TABLE OF CONTENTS

- Weight Management

- Eating for Heart Health, Bone Health, and More

Chapter 5: Special Diets and Dietary Restrictions

- Vegetarianism and Veganism

- Gluten-Free and Dairy-Free Diets

- Managing Food Allergies

Chapter 6: Meal Planning and Preparation

- Creating Nutrient-Dense Meals

- Smart Shopping and Budget-Friendly Choices

- Cooking Tips and Techniques

Chapter 7: Diet Trends and Fads

- Evaluating Popular Diets (Keto, Paleo, Intermittent Fasting)

- Debunking Nutrition Myths

- The Importance of Sustainable Eating Habits

Chapter 8: Nutrition Throughout the Lifespan

- Nutrition for Children and Adolescents

- Eating Well During Pregnancy and Breastfeeding

- Senior Nutrition and Aging Gracefully

Introduction

" This eBook is your comprehensive guide to understanding the intricacies of nutrition and harnessing the power of food to enhance your vitality, support your health goals, and elevate your quality of life.

In the pages that follow, we embark on a journey through the fascinating landscape of nutrition, demystifying the science behind the foods we consume. We will explore the essential macronutrients and micronutrients, delve into the inner workings of your digestive system, and uncover the profound impact of diet on your health.

Whether you're a seasoned health enthusiast, a novice looking to make better dietary choices, or simply curious about the role of nutrition in your life, this eBook has something to offer. We'll cover everything from the basics of a balanced diet to specialized eating plans, all with the aim of empowering you to make informed decisions about what you put on your plate.

Along the way, you'll discover practical tips for meal planning, navigating the challenges of dietary restrictions, and adopting sustainable eating habits that can stand the test of time. We'll also delve into the role of nutrition in different life stages, from childhood to the golden years, and explore how it impacts your athletic performance and overall well-being.

As we traverse the evolving landscape of nutrition in the modern world, we'll address the intersection of technology, sustainability, and dietary choices. Together, we'll learn how to make mindful decisions about what we eat, not just for our personal health but also for the health of the planet.

Chapter 1: The Fundamentals of Nutrition

Imagine your body as a finely tuned machine, and the food you eat as the fuel that keeps it running. Just as a car requires the right type of fuel to operate efficiently, your body relies on specific nutrients to function optimally.

Understanding Macronutrients and Micronutrients

At the heart of nutrition are two key categories of nutrients: macronutrients and micronutrients.

Macronutrients are the primary sources of energy for your body. They consist of:

1. Carbohydrates: Often misunderstood and unfairly demonized, carbohydrates are your body's preferred source of energy. They come in two main forms: simple carbohydrates (found in foods like sugars and fruit) and complex carbohydrates (found in grains, legumes, and vegetables). The key is to choose complex carbs for sustained energy.

2. Proteins: Proteins are the building blocks of life. They play a crucial role in repairing tissues, building muscle, and supporting various bodily functions. Sources of protein include meat, poultry, fish, dairy products, beans, and tofu.

3. Fats: Fats are essential for overall health. They provide energy, help absorb fat-soluble vitamins, and contribute to the structure of cell membranes. Healthy fats, such as those found in avocados, nuts, and olive oil, should be a part of your diet.

Micronutrients are the vitamins and minerals that your body requires in smaller quantities but are no less important. They are involved in various biochemical processes and play vital roles in maintaining good health. Some examples include:

- Vitamins: These organic compounds are needed for various functions, such as vitamin C for a robust immune system and vitamin D for bone health. They can be found in a variety of foods, and a balanced diet typically provides all the vitamins you need.

- Minerals: Minerals like calcium, magnesium, and potassium are essential for bone health, muscle function, and maintaining proper fluid balance in the body. Sources of minerals range from dairy products to leafy greens.

The Role of Water in Nutrition

While often overlooked, water is arguably the most critical nutrient of all. Your body is composed of roughly 60% water, and it's involved in nearly every bodily function. Water helps regulate body temperature, transport nutrients, and remove waste products. Staying adequately hydrated is vital for overall health.

As you embark on your journey to better nutrition, keep these fundamental concepts in mind. Macronutrients and micronutrients are the building blocks of a healthy diet, and understanding their roles will empower you to make informed choices about the foods you consume.

Chapter 2: The Science of Digestion

In our journey to understand nutrition, we must venture beyond what we eat and explore how our bodies process the foods we consume. This chapter delves into the intricate world of digestion, shedding light on the fascinating processes that transform your meals into the energy and nutrients your body needs to thrive.

How Your Body Processes Food

Digestion is a complex and highly coordinated process that begins the moment you take your first bite. Here's a simplified overview of how your body processes food:

1. Mouth: Digestion begins in your mouth, where enzymes in your saliva start breaking down carbohydrates. Chewing your food thoroughly aids this process.

2. Esophagus: Once you swallow, food travels down the esophagus and into the stomach through a muscular tube called the esophagus.

3. Stomach: In the stomach, food encounters gastric juices that contain hydrochloric acid and enzymes. These chemicals help break down proteins and kill harmful bacteria.

4. Small Intestine: The partially digested food then moves into the small intestine, where most of the nutrient absorption occurs. Enzymes from the pancreas and bile from the liver further aid digestion.

5. Absorption: Nutrients, now in their smaller forms, are absorbed into the bloodstream through the walls of the small intestine. Carbohydrates turn into sugars, proteins into amino acids, and fats into fatty acids.

6. Large Intestine: What's left after absorption enters the large intestine, where water and some minerals are absorbed. The remaining material is eventually eliminated as waste.

The Digestive System's Key Players

Several organs and structures play essential roles in the digestive process:

- Pancreas: Produces digestive enzymes and hormones like insulin.

- Liver: Produces bile, which emulsifies fats to aid digestion.

- Gallbladder: Stores and releases bile into the small intestine when needed.

- Small Intestine: The site of most nutrient absorption.

- Large Intestine (Colon): Where water and some minerals are absorbed, and waste is formed.

Understanding this journey from mouth to large intestine is crucial because it highlights the importance of efficient digestion. Your body relies on this process to extract the nutrients it needs to function correctly.

Absorption and Metabolism

Once nutrients are absorbed into the bloodstream, they become the building blocks and energy sources your body uses. Carbohydrates provide energy, proteins support tissue repair, and fats serve as an energy reserve. The absorbed nutrients are transported to cells throughout the body, where they participate in countless biochemical reactions.

Metabolism, the sum of these chemical processes, ensures that nutrients are used for energy, growth, and repair. A well-functioning metabolism is essential for maintaining a healthy weight and overall well-being.

By understanding the science of digestion, you'll gain valuable insights into how to optimize your diet for better health and vitality.

Chapter 3: Balancing Your Diet

In our exploration of nutrition, we've covered the basics of nutrients and the intricate science of digestion. Now, it's time to delve into a crucial aspect of maintaining good health - the art of balancing your diet.

Building a Balanced Plate

A balanced diet is like a symphony of nutrients, where each plays a harmonious role in promoting your overall well-being. To achieve this balance, it's helpful to visualize your plate as a canvas, with different food groups coming together to create a masterpiece of nutrition.

Here's how you can build a balanced plate:

1. Fruits and Vegetables: Fill half your plate with a colorful array of fruits and vegetables. They are rich in vitamins, minerals, fiber, and antioxidants. Aim for a variety of colors and types to ensure you get a broad spectrum of nutrients.

2. Proteins: Include a moderate portion of lean proteins, such as poultry, fish, tofu, beans, or legumes. Protein is essential for muscle maintenance, repair, and overall body function.

3. Grains: Choose whole grains like brown rice, quinoa, whole wheat pasta, and oats. Whole grains are a source of complex carbohydrates and fiber, providing long-lasting energy and digestive health benefits.

4. Healthy Fats: Incorporate sources of healthy fats, such as avocados, nuts, seeds, and olive oil. These fats support brain function, hormone production, and the absorption of fat-soluble vitamins.

5. Dairy or Dairy Alternatives: If you consume dairy, opt for low-fat or non-fat options. Alternatively, choose dairy-free alternatives like almond milk or soy yogurt if you're lactose intolerant or prefer plant-based options.

6. Portion Control: Be mindful of portion sizes. Overeating, even healthy foods, can lead to excess calorie intake. Use smaller plates to help control portions.

Portion Control and Serving Sizes

Understanding portion control is vital to maintaining a balanced diet and managing your weight. Here are some tips to help you control portion sizes:

- Use visual cues: A serving of protein is about the size of your palm, a cupped hand equals one serving of grains, and a fist is roughly the size of a serving of vegetables.

- Read labels: Nutrition labels on packaged foods provide information on serving sizes and calories per serving. Pay attention to these details when choosing your portions.

- Listen to your body: Pay attention to hunger and fullness cues. Eat slowly, savoring each bite, and stop when you're satisfied, not overly full.

Dietary Guidelines for Health

Many countries provide dietary guidelines to help individuals make informed choices about their diet. These guidelines typically recommend:

- Balancing calories: Maintain a balance between the calories you consume and those you expend through physical activity.

- Choosing nutrient-dense foods: Prioritize foods rich in nutrients and limit empty-calorie options.

- Limiting added sugars and salt: Reduce your intake of foods and beverages high in added sugars and sodium.

- Being mindful of portion sizes: Control portion sizes to avoid overeating.

- Balancing food groups: Consume a variety of foods from all food groups to ensure a well-rounded diet.

Balancing your diet is not about strict rules or deprivation; it's about making choices that support your health and well-being. By creating a balanced plate and being mindful of portion sizes, you can harness the power of nutrition to nourish your body for a healthier, happier life.

Chapter 4: The Impact of Diet on Health

In this chapter, we venture deep into the heart of the matter—the profound impact of your dietary choices on your health and well-being. It's no exaggeration to say that what you eat can determine your quality of life. From preventing chronic diseases to boosting your energy levels, your diet plays a central role in your overall health.

The Link Between Diet and Chronic Diseases

Chronic diseases, such as heart disease, type 2 diabetes, and certain cancers, have reached epidemic proportions in many parts of the world. It's essential to understand that many of these diseases are closely linked to diet and lifestyle factors.

- Heart Disease: High intake of saturated and trans fats, along with excess salt and sugar, can contribute to heart disease. On the other hand, diets rich in fruits, vegetables, and whole grains can help reduce the risk.

- Type 2 Diabetes: Poor dietary choices, including excessive consumption of sugary and processed foods, can increase the risk of developing type 2 diabetes. Balanced diets with controlled sugar intake can help manage and prevent this condition.

- Cancer: While cancer is a complex disease with various risk factors, diet plays a crucial role. Consuming a diet high in fruits and vegetables with cancer-fighting compounds can lower the risk.

Weight Management and Obesity

Obesity is a growing global health concern. It's often a result of an imbalance between the calories you consume and those you expend. This chapter discusses how dietary choices, portion control, and mindful eating can aid in weight management. It also emphasizes the importance of sustainable, long-term approaches to weight loss and maintenance.

Eating for Specific Health Goals

Your diet can be tailored to meet specific health goals, whether it's improving heart health, managing blood pressure, or supporting bone health. Explore how adjusting your diet to address these goals can have a transformative impact on your well-being.

Mindful Eating and Emotional Eating

Mindful eating involves paying attention to your food, savoring each bite, and listening to your body's hunger and fullness cues. We'll delve into the concept of mindful eating and provide strategies to overcome emotional eating, which can lead to unhealthy food choices.

The Power of Prevention

The saying, "an ounce of prevention is worth a pound of cure," rings especially true in the realm of nutrition. By adopting a diet rich in nutrient-dense foods, minimizing processed and sugary options, and staying hydrated, you can significantly reduce your risk of chronic diseases.

In the following chapters, we'll delve into practical strategies for implementing a healthier diet, including meal planning, understanding dietary restrictions, and exploring the latest trends in nutrition. Armed with knowledge about the profound impact of diet on health, you'll be better equipped to make informed choices that promote a long and healthy life.

Chapter 5: Special Diets and Dietary Restrictions

In the diverse landscape of nutrition, there exists a myriad of dietary choices and restrictions. This chapter explores various special diets and dietary restrictions, shedding light on why people adopt them and how to navigate these nutritional paths while maintaining health and well-being.

The Rise of Special Diets

Special diets have gained popularity for a variety of reasons, ranging from ethical beliefs to health concerns and food intolerances. Here, we'll delve into some of the most prevalent special diets and discuss the motivations behind them.

Vegetarianism and Veganism

- Vegetarianism: Vegetarians abstain from consuming meat, poultry, and fish while incorporating plant-based foods into their diet. Learn about the different types of vegetarians, from lacto-vegetarians to ovo-vegetarians.

- Veganism: Vegans take plant-based eating a step further by eliminating all animal products, including dairy, eggs, and honey, from their diet. Discover the ethical, environmental, and health reasons behind choosing a vegan lifestyle.

Gluten-Free and Dairy-Free Diets

- Gluten-Free Diet: Individuals with celiac disease or gluten sensitivity must avoid gluten-containing grains like wheat, barley, and rye. We'll explore the intricacies of gluten-free living and provide guidance for those with gluten-related disorders.

- **Dairy-Free Diet**: Lactose intolerance and dairy allergies are common reasons for avoiding dairy products. This section discusses dairy-free alternatives and ensuring adequate calcium intake.

Managing Food Allergies

- Food Allergies: Food allergies can be life-threatening, and individuals with allergies must vigilantly avoid allergens. We'll cover common allergens, label reading, and allergen-safe food preparation.

Paleo and Keto Diets

- Paleo Diet: The paleolithic diet mimics the presumed eating habits of our ancestors. It emphasizes whole foods, lean proteins, and the exclusion of grains and processed foods.

- Ketogenic Diet (Keto): The keto diet is low in carbohydrates and high in fats, designed to induce a state of ketosis. We'll discuss the science behind ketosis and the potential benefits and drawbacks of this diet.

Navigating Special Diets and Dietary Restrictions

Successfully adopting a special diet or adhering to dietary restrictions requires careful planning and consideration of nutritional needs. We'll provide practical tips for ensuring that you get all the essential nutrients while following your chosen dietary path.

Balancing Special Diets with Health Goals

It's crucial to align your special diet with your health goals. Whether you're striving for weight loss, improved heart health, or ethical choices, we'll guide you on how to optimize your chosen diet to meet your objectives.

Chapter 6: Meal Planning and Preparation

In the quest for better nutrition, the choices you make in the kitchen play a pivotal role. Chapter 6 is all about empowering you with the knowledge and skills to plan and prepare nutritious meals that align with your health and dietary goals.

The Benefits of Meal Planning

Meal planning isn't just about convenience; it's a strategic tool that can help you make healthier food choices, save time, reduce food waste, and stay on budget. Here, we'll explore the many advantages of meal planning.

Creating Balanced and Nutrient-Dense Meals

Meal planning starts with a well-balanced plate. We'll delve into the principles of creating balanced meals that include a variety of foods from different food groups. Discover how to incorporate the essential macronutrients and micronutrients into your daily meals.

Portion Control and Mindful Eating

Overeating is a common challenge when it comes to maintaining a healthy diet. Learn how portion control can help you manage your calorie intake and prevent overindulgence. Additionally, we'll explore the concept of mindful eating, which encourages a deeper connection with your food and listening to your body's hunger and fullness cues.

Smart Shopping for Success

Effective meal planning begins at the grocery store. We'll provide tips for smart shopping, including creating a shopping list, reading food labels, and choosing fresh, whole foods. These strategies can help you make nutritious choices while avoiding the temptations of less healthy options.

Meal Prep Techniques

Meal prep is a time-saving practice that involves preparing ingredients or even full meals in advance. We'll discuss different meal prep techniques, from batch cooking to assembling freezer-friendly meals. With the right approach, you can have healthy meals ready at a moment's notice.

Cooking Tips and Techniques

Cooking need not be intimidating. We'll cover basic cooking techniques and tips that can turn anyone into a confident home cook. From sautéing and roasting to steaming and grilling, you'll gain the skills needed to prepare delicious, wholesome meals.

Special Considerations: Dietary Restrictions and Preferences

If you have dietary restrictions or specific preferences, meal planning can be tailored to suit your needs. We'll explore how to adapt meal planning for vegetarian, vegan, gluten-free, or other specialized diets.

Meal Planning Tools and Resources

To simplify the meal planning process, we'll introduce you to various tools and resources, including meal planning apps, websites, and cookbooks. These resources can assist you in creating balanced, enjoyable, and health-conscious meal plans.

Chapter 7: Diet Trends and Fads

In the ever-evolving landscape of nutrition, diet trends and fads come and go, each promising transformative results. In this chapter, we'll embark on a journey through some of the most popular diet trends, providing insight into their principles, potential benefits, and the importance of critical thinking when evaluating their suitability for your health and lifestyle.

Understanding Diet Trends

Diet trends can capture our attention with alluring promises of rapid weight loss, increased energy, or better health. However, it's essential to approach these trends with a discerning eye. In this section, we'll explore the reasons behind the popularity of diet trends and the psychology that drives our fascination with them.

The Keto Diet

The ketogenic diet, or "keto" for short, has gained immense popularity in recent years. It involves drastically reducing carbohydrates and replacing them with fats, aiming to induce a state of ketosis where the body burns fat for energy. We'll delve into the science behind keto, its potential benefits, and considerations for those considering this high-fat, low-carb approach.

The Paleo Diet

The paleolithic diet, often referred to as the "paleo" diet, seeks to mimic the eating habits of our ancient ancestors. It emphasizes whole foods, lean proteins, and the avoidance of grains, legumes, and processed foods. We'll explore the principles of the paleo diet and its potential benefits and drawbacks.

Intermittent Fasting

Intermittent fasting (IF) involves cycling between periods of eating and fasting. It has garnered attention for its potential weight loss and metabolic benefits. We'll discuss the various forms of intermittent fasting and explore the science and practical aspects of this eating pattern.

Plant-Based Diets

Plant-based diets, including vegetarianism and veganism, have seen increased adoption due to ethical, environmental, and health concerns. We'll examine the motivations behind plant-based diets, their potential health benefits, and strategies for meeting nutrient needs while following these dietary choices.

The Importance of Sustainable Eating Habits

While diet trends may offer short-term benefits, sustainability and long-term adherence are key to maintaining a healthy diet. We'll emphasize the importance of finding dietary choices that align with your lifestyle, values, and overall well-being.

Evaluating Diet Trends Critically

Critical thinking is essential when evaluating diet trends. We'll provide a framework for assessing diet trends, considering factors such as scientific evidence, individual needs, and long-term feasibility. This empowers you to make informed decisions about whether a particular trend is suitable for you.

Chapter 8: Nutrition Throughout the Lifespan

In this chapter, we embark on a journey through the stages of life, exploring how nutrition plays a vital role in promoting health and well-being from childhood through adolescence, into adulthood, and during the golden years of seniority.

Nutrition in Early Life: Infancy and Childhood

The foundation of good health is laid in infancy and childhood. We'll discuss the importance of breastfeeding, introducing solid foods, and promoting a varied diet rich in essential nutrients during these formative years. Proper nutrition in childhood supports growth, development, and sets the stage for lifelong habits.

Adolescent Nutrition: Navigating Growth and Change

Adolescence is a time of rapid growth and change. We'll explore the unique nutritional needs of teenagers, including the increased demand for energy, calcium, and iron. We'll also discuss strategies for addressing common dietary challenges faced by adolescents.

Adult Nutrition: Supporting a Busy Life

In adulthood, busy schedules and responsibilities can sometimes lead to dietary neglect. We'll provide guidance on maintaining a balanced diet while juggling work, family, and social commitments. We'll also discuss the role of nutrition in managing stress, weight, and overall health.

Nutrition During Pregnancy and Breastfeeding

Pregnancy is a unique and transformative period for women. We'll delve into the dietary needs of expectant mothers, highlighting the importance of prenatal nutrition and discussing key nutrients like folic acid, iron, and calcium. We'll also explore breastfeeding and its benefits for both mother and baby.

Nutrition in the Senior Years: Aging Gracefully

As we age, our nutritional needs evolve. We'll discuss the dietary considerations for older adults, including maintaining bone health, managing chronic conditions, and adapting to changes in metabolism. We'll also emphasize the importance of hydration and a balanced diet in supporting the aging process.

Lifelong Healthy Eating Habits

Throughout these life stages, the cultivation of healthy eating habits remains essential. We'll provide strategies for maintaining a nutritious diet throughout life, including portion control, mindful eating, and adapting to changing dietary needs.

Chapter 9: Sports Nutrition

In this chapter, we'll dive into the fascinating world of sports nutrition, where the relationship between what you eat and how you perform is paramount. Whether you're an elite athlete or someone who enjoys staying active, understanding the role of nutrition in sports can help you optimize your performance and recovery.

The Importance of Sports Nutrition

Proper nutrition can be the difference between reaching your athletic goals and falling short. We'll explore why sports nutrition matters and how it can positively impact your physical performance, endurance, and recovery.

Macronutrients for Athletic Success

Athletes have unique macronutrient needs. We'll discuss the role of carbohydrates, proteins, and fats in providing energy, supporting muscle growth and repair, and ensuring stamina during workouts and competitions.

Hydration and Electrolyte Balance

Staying hydrated is critical for athletes. We'll delve into the importance of proper hydration, especially during physical activity, and explore the role of electrolytes in maintaining fluid balance and muscle function.

Timing Your Nutrition

The timing of your meals and snacks can significantly impact your performance. We'll discuss pre-exercise, during-exercise, and post-exercise nutrition strategies to help you maximize your workouts and enhance recovery.

Supplements in Sports Nutrition

Supplements are a hot topic in the world of sports nutrition. We'll provide insights into common supplements used by athletes, including protein powders, creatine, and branched-chain amino acids. We'll also emphasize the importance of using supplements wisely and under professional guidance.

Eating for Endurance vs. Strength

Different sports require different nutritional approaches. We'll distinguish between endurance sports, which demand sustained energy, and strength-based activities, which focus on muscle development. You'll learn how to tailor your diet to your specific athletic pursuits.

Meal Planning for Athletes

Athletes need to eat strategically. We'll offer practical meal planning tips and sample meal ideas for before, during, and after exercise. Whether you're training for a marathon or hitting the gym, these meal plans can help you fuel up effectively.

Recovery Nutrition

Recovery is an often-overlooked aspect of sports nutrition. We'll discuss the importance of post-exercise nutrition for muscle repair and glycogen replenishment, along with strategies to promote a quicker recovery.

By the end of this chapter, you'll have a solid understanding of how nutrition impacts athletic performance and the tools to optimize your diet for your specific sports and fitness goals. Whether you're a competitive athlete or someone who enjoys staying active, the principles of sports nutrition can help you reach your peak potential.

Chapter 10: Nutrition in a Modern World

In this chapter, we'll navigate the complex landscape of nutrition in a rapidly changing modern world. We'll explore the impact of technology, food marketing, and lifestyle choices on our dietary habits, as well as the importance of mindful eating and sustainable practices.

The Influence of Technology

Technology has reshaped the way we approach nutrition. We'll discuss how smart phones, apps, and wearable devices have revolutionized tracking and monitoring of dietary choices, calorie intake, and physical activity. We'll also examine the benefits and potential pitfalls of relying on technology for nutrition guidance.

Food Marketing and Label Reading

Food marketing is pervasive, and understanding its influence is crucial. We'll delve into how marketing strategies can sway our food choices and provide insights into reading food labels critically. Armed with this knowledge, you can make informed decisions at the grocery store.

Eating on the Go

Modern life often leaves little time for leisurely meals. We'll explore the challenges of eating on the go and offer practical strategies for making nutritious choices when dining out or grabbing meals during a busy day

The Role of Convenience Foods

Convenience foods have become a staple of modern diets. We'll discuss the impact of processed and fast foods on health and provide guidance on how to make healthier choices when convenience is a necessity.

Mindful Eating: A Counterbalance to Modern Rush

Mindful eating is a practice that encourages you to be present in the moment while eating, paying full attention to your food and the act of eating itself. We'll explore the benefits of mindful eating, including improved digestion, better portion control, and a healthier relationship with food.

Sustainable Eating Practices

The modern world's demand for food has environmental consequences. We'll delve into the concept of sustainable eating, which involves making choices that are both healthy for you and the planet. We'll discuss reducing food waste, choosing locally sourced foods, and the benefits of a plant-based diet for sustainability.

Building a Balanced Diet in a Modern World

Balancing nutrition in a fast-paced, technology-driven world can be challenging, but it's essential for long-term health and well-being. We'll provide practical strategies for building and maintaining a balanced diet, even amidst the demands of modern life.

Chapter 11: Building Healthy Habits

In this chapter, we'll explore the power of habits in shaping our dietary choices and overall well-being. We'll delve into the science of habit formation, offer practical strategies for building and maintaining healthy eating habits, and discuss the role of consistency in long-term success.

Understanding the Science of Habits

Habits are the building blocks of our daily routines, and they have a profound impact on our lives. We'll explore the science of habit formation, including how habits are developed, maintained, and altered. Understanding this process is key to making lasting changes in your eating habits.

The Habit Loop: Cue, Routine, Reward

Habits follow a loop: cue, routine, reward. We'll break down this loop, helping you identify the cues that trigger your eating habits, the routines themselves, and the rewards you seek. Recognizing these components is the first step in modifying or creating new habits.

Replacing Unhealthy Habits with Healthy Ones

If you have unhealthy eating habits, you're not alone. We'll provide practical strategies for replacing these habits with healthier alternatives. Whether it's reducing sugary snacks, late-night eating, or excessive caffeine consumption, we'll guide you through the process of change.

The Power of Goal Setting

Setting clear and achievable goals is a critical part of habit formation. We'll discuss the importance of goal setting in building healthy eating habits, including how to create SMART (Specific, Measurable, Achievable, Relevant, and Time-bound) goals that motivate and guide your progress.

Meal Planning as a Habit

Meal planning and preparation can become habitual, making it easier to maintain a balanced diet. We'll revisit the meal planning strategies discussed earlier in the eBook and show how they can be integrated into your daily routine.

Consistency and Resilience

Consistency is the backbone of habit formation. We'll explore the role of consistency in building and maintaining healthy eating habits, along with strategies for staying on track even when faced with challenges and setbacks.

Mindful Eating as a Daily Practice

Mindful eating isn't just an occasional practice; it can become a daily habit. We'll revisit the concept of mindful eating and discuss how incorporating it into your meals can lead to healthier, more enjoyable eating experiences.

Building a Lifetime of Healthy Eating Habits

Building healthy eating habits isn't a temporary endeavor; it's a lifelong journey. We'll discuss the importance of viewing habits as a long-term commitment and provide guidance on maintaining the progress you've made.

Conclusion

Conclusion

In this final chapter, we reflect on the journey we've taken through the world of nutrition and diet. We'll summarize key takeaways, offer guidance for sustaining your newfound knowledge, and inspire you to embrace a future of lifelong health and wellness.

Recap of Key Takeaways

Before we move forward, let's revisit some of the essential lessons we've explored throughout this eBook:

- The profound impact of diet on health and well-being.

- Understanding macronutrients, micronutrients, and their roles.

- The importance of balanced meals and portion control.

- Special diets, dietary restrictions, and dietary preferences.

- The significance of meal planning and preparation.

- Evaluating and critically assessing diet trends and fads.

- Nutrition's role throughout different life stages.

- Navigating the modern world of technology and convenience.

- Building and maintaining healthy eating habits.

Your Personalized Nutrition Blueprint

Now that you've acquired knowledge, it's time to create your personalized nutrition blueprint. Consider your individual goals, dietary preferences, and any specific health concerns you may have. This blueprint will serve as your guide for making informed dietary choices that align with your unique needs.

Sustaining Lifelong Wellness

The journey to better nutrition doesn't end with this eBook. It's a lifelong pursuit of health and wellness. Here are some tips to help you sustain your commitment to a healthier future:

1.   Continuous Learning: Nutrition is a dynamic field. Stay curious and keep learning about the latest research, trends, and developments in nutrition and dietary science.

2.   Regular Check-Ins: Periodically assess your dietary choices and habits to ensure they align with your goals. Adjust as needed to maintain balance and well-being.

3.   Stay Mindful: Continue practicing mindful eating, paying attention to your body's hunger and fullness cues, and savoring each meal.

4. Supportive Community: Surround yourself with a community of like-minded individuals who share your commitment to health. Sharing experiences and tips can provide motivation and accountability.

5.   Seek Professional Guidance: When in doubt or facing specific health challenges, consult with a registered dietitian or healthcare professional for personalized guidance and support.

6. Balance and Variety: Maintain a diverse and balanced diet. Explore different cuisines and foods to keep your meals exciting and nutrient-rich.

7. Physical Activity: Remember that diet is only one piece of the puzzle. Regular physical activity is equally crucial for overall health and well-being.

Embracing a Healthier Future

As you move forward on your nutritional journey, remember that it's not about perfection but progress. Embrace the knowledge and habits you've gained, and let them guide you toward a healthier and happier future.

Your commitment to better nutrition is an investment in your well-being, vitality, and longevity. With the tools and insights you've acquired in this eBook, you have the power to make informed choices, overcome challenges, and create a life filled with health, vitality, and joy.